To
Noah

...mee

MEMOIRS

Look forward to

OF *hearing your story*

DOCTOR DOG

OLD-FASHIONED TALES

FROM A VETERINARIAN

DR. BRUCE KEENE

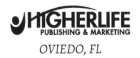

HIGHERLIFE
PUBLISHING & MARKETING

OVIEDO, FL

HigherLife Publishing & Marketing
PO Box 623307
Oviedo, FL 32762
AHigherLife.com

Memoirs of Doctor Dog/ Dr. Bruce Keene -- 1st ed.
ISBN 978-1-951492-45-8 Paperback
ISBN 978-1-951492-46-5 eBook

Contents

Part 1: Life Lessons

Part II: The College Years

Part III: Veterinary Practice Work

Part IV: Joining Forces in Veterinary Medicine

Part V: Final Stories

Personally, I have always felt that the best doctor in the world is the Veterinarian. He can't ask his patients what is the matter...he's just got to know.

—WILL ROGERS

MY ORIGINAL TARGET AUDIENCE for this book was other veterinarians, vet techs, and compassionate animal lovers. I began writing this book for the people that have told me they aspired to be a veterinarian and for all the young students that still do.

It should be read as entertainment as I share stories from my 55 years of practice as a veterinarian. I have seen the evolution of the profession of veterinary medicine from my work taking care of cows to dogs and how small practices work in contrast to corporate-specialty practices. I have also lived through the dissolution of the family farm, the changing educational landscape from men to women in vet school, and the end of the greyhound racing industry in the state of Florida. I believe that sharing these changes is of historical significance to my profession. My wife of 60 years, who is a PhD, has helped me to understand the relationship called the human-animal bond and the human-personality, both of which shaped the changes to my care as a veterinarian.

During the process of editing these memoirs, the editor mentioned that there were many sad stories. Three of these stories occurred during my early internship in Magnolia, Arkansas. One resulted from bad advice from another vet. The other experiences occurred during my 30 years at Lake Howell Animal Hospital.

The truth is that life is tragic, especially as a vet. Most of the stories in this collection are not sad, but rather serendipitous as they had great benefit to my career along with the gift of God's grace. Throughout my journey as a vet, I have learned a lot about life and animals. Here are a few of those important insights:

- I learned about the humane treatment of animals as it relates to euthanasia.
- I learned to counsel clients in their grief in the loss of a family pet.
- I learned how to answer the question, "Do animals go to heaven?"
- I learned about the spirituality of the human-animal relationship.
- I learned about my personal spirituality and my faith.

I dedicate this book with thanksgiving for my great mentors and the important things that life as a veterinarian has taught me about faith, love, and happiness. Enjoy!

PART I
LIFE LESSONS

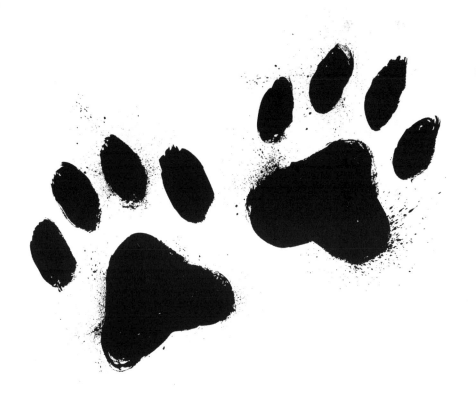

CHAPTER 1

Growing Up

MY FATHER CHANGED JOBS several times during my elementary school years finally settling down to work as an accountant for the state highway department. Each move created a lot of stress for me because I had to start over in a new school and create new friendships. During my junior and high school years, both of my parents worked hard at their jobs, but the last few years things changed toward an unhappy marriage. They had many fights, with my mother defending us against my fathers' evening drinking, temper, and sometimes excessive punishment. I remember experiencing quite a bit of his "belt discipline." They admitted they were "just staying together for the kids' sake." These experiences resulted in my becoming fearful of my father and looking forward to leaving home. For me, my fathers' life philosophy seemed to be that success in life was measured by how smart a child was in math. Since my younger brother had more of Dad's personality and was brighter in math, he seemed to have my fathers' favor and blessing. On the other hand, I developed a phobia of math from his pressure. This resulted in my avoidance of any math related subject. Without encouragement, I had a low self-esteem and didn't think I was very smart. I'll never forget the crisis I had in the 9th grade. Following another family move and change of schools, I met two bullies. The first was a geometry teacher. He loved to call on the scared, nervous students, like myself to come to the front of the room and humiliate them by solving math problems on the black board. Of course, with my math phobia and low confidence at the time, I dreaded that class the most. To make matters worse, in that same class there was a class bully who was constantly trying to pick a fight with me. I really feared the school's disciplinary action and my father's later punishment more than the fight. I remember having great anxiety each morning before school started. I appreciated a friend who would kindly walk with me around the school block to calm my nervousness for the day.

Another experience with a bully that added to my school insecurities at that time came in football. I have always liked sports and outdoor activities. As such, I decided to go out for the football team. Unfortunately, the coach was another intimidating bully. I had no previous experience playing football and he didn't have patience with me or time to teach me. Instead, when I missed my first blocking assignment, physically attacked me, cursing me, and knocking me to the ground. Since I had enough of that at home, I quit. To this day, I regret that I did not get a chance to play football.

However, I am thankful I joined the school track team and became our school's primary pole vaulter/ high jumper. This was an important step in giving me the boost I needed for my confidence. I continued to do well in vaulting throughout high school, being ranked in the top three in the state. This track success resulted in being esteemed by my classmates.

I also became a reporter for our school paper. I once wrote an article humorously pointing out the virtues of having big feet called, "Shorty's Sad Shoe Story" as my feet are a size 13! I found this action of turning my embarrassment into a positive helped a lot.

I am the oldest son of four children. My siblings include a younger brother and a pair of twins – a brother and a sister. As the oldest, I had to set the example for the other children.

In the early days of my boyhood, our family had some happy times. I remember with my parent's dual income, they were able to build a new home, buy a new Buick car, and provide us with nice Christmas gifts. I was proud of our new home and overseeing finding a Christmas tree for us each year. I was my mother's handyman. One year, I even built a play dresser gift for my sister.

To my father's credit, he did require my brother and me to work paper routes for two years to save for college. We believe that working on our paper routes helped teach us valuable skills that have helped us as entrepreneurs.

For example, on my 120-customer paper route, I had three distinct residential areas to cover. This route was on a very hilly part of Little Rock, Arkansas requiring a lot of mountain biking. In the first area, the homes were older, modest, working class, smaller homes. In the second area, the homes were new and built for the middle class. These were built with a hilltop view of the valley where we lived. The last area of homes were the large estate mansions built upon a mountain top along the skyline of the Arkansas River. I had to pedal my bike down long driveways to put the paper on these "rich people's" porches. I looked forward to a nice Christmas gift for my effort. Sadly, I did not receive anything. Instead the customers that gave me food and gifts at Christmas were the working class in the first group of homes.

Another lesson I learned was during the collection of monthly bills. Of course, the newspaper company was always paid first and then it was my responsibility to collect my profit from what was left. The customers were hard to catch at home and the no-pay accounts came out of my pocket. After a couple years, my brother and I were able to save over $1000 each for our college education. I remember, my father's only business advice was, "It's a cold, cold business world out there."

DR. BRUCE KEENE

CHAPTER 2

Understanding Relationships & Human Personalities

GOD HAS BLESSED ME with 59 years of marriage to my wife, Barbara. She has always been my biggest supporter. For instance, she always believed in me becoming a veterinarian when I had a lot of doubt. During our first years of marriage, she financially supported us by working as a schoolteacher. Later, I supported her going back to college and earning her master's degree and PhD in Mental Health Counseling. I believe that her study of Psychology helped me learn a lot about our marriage, myself, and my father-son relationship.

One test she used when counseling her clients was the Myers-Briggs personality profile. This test classifies individuals in four areas of personality types. According to the test, people are classified as either Extroverts or Introverts, as Sensory or Intuitive, Feeling or Thinking, and Judgmental or Perceiving.

During some of our early experiences with small church groups, we learned most marriages are attracted to opposite partners in the personality profile. This can work for us or against us. For instance, my wife is an extrovert, intuitive, feeling, perceiving person, liking spontaneity. I am a conservative, introverted, sensory, logical thinker, very structured and organized. By making this difference an asset, rather than a source of conflict, it has helped us survive nearly 60 years of marriage.

Regarding my father's personality, I remember he used to love having lengthy morning conversations over coffee with my wife. In personality, they were much alike. My father once told me as a boy, he just didn't understand me. I now know that was because we were different. His personality was also much like my brother. For instance, my brother would stand up to my father and our football coach's strong discipline. I, on other hand, avoided conflict at all cost. I remember my father perceived this as weakness in me and my mother always wanted me to stand up to his "belt" punishment.

Later in my veterinary reading of animal behavior, one book I read really helped my father-son relationship. In *Horse Sense for Humans*, written by Marty

Roberts, who is known as the "horse whisperer," Marty teaches horses to accept a saddle through encouragement and gaining their trust. He calls it "joining up." This method helps the horses overcome their fears of predators like cougars. Through his method of "gentle training," a horse they will accept a saddle in half the time as the old method seen in rodeos of the saddleback bucking method, which involves breaking them into submission.

Marty explains that there are two types of teachers in life. The first are extrinsic teachers, meaning that they teach from the outside as an authority or intimidator. These are like the rodeo cowboys. In my life, my father would be this type. The second type are the intrinsic teachers, like the horse whisperer, who teach by encouragement. Marty also teaches business communication skills using his animal methods in the human corporate world.

In the book, *The Shack*, a father-son relationship similar to my own was healed by forgiveness and the relationship with God and Jesus. I had that same healing experience with my faith walk and the understanding of how my father's parenting methods were helpful to me.

In this book, the author also says the father-son relationship is powerful and all sons want to be loved and blessed by their fathers. He thinks the spirit is enormously important. In teaching slowly and patiently, he says results are achieved faster.

Another animal related book that helped me a lot was *Thinking in Pictures* by Temple Grandin. Grandin, who is autistic, teaches that there are two types of communicators in life. The first are verbal communicators, like my wife and my father, as they use words to communicate. The second are sensory communicators, like Ms. Grandin and I. We are visual, analytical, solitary, religious thinkers. We are the more sensitive and feeling-type personalities.

Animals like horses and cattle are sensory communicators. They think in pictures. They rely on a memory library of past experiences. Grandin has used her understanding of autism in the cattle industry to redesign slaughterhouses all over the county. Thinking from the animal's fearful prospective is more humane and reduces stress, injury, and disease, which results in better production in the animals.

Overall, the experiences, intimidators, and bullies in my life have taught me great things. And later, in my pre-vet college course work, an intrinsic Physics professor taught me how to overcome my math phobia. As such, one of my proudest accomplishments in college was earning a B in Physics.

Another proud accomplishment in my life was passing the difficult instrument rating qualifying test as a pilot with another intrinsic teacher. Besides healing my father-son relationship, this teacher helped me overcome my fear of math and later answered my prayer to become a veterinarian.

DR. BRUCE KEENE

CHAPTER 3

Life on the Farm

My mother was raised on an 80-acre dairy farm in Minnesota. Each summer, my younger brother and I would spend our summer school vacations on that farm.

I had a special, quiet place in a treehouse out in the pasture behind their barn there. On a regular basis, I would climb up there to dream about my future. I now relate that to the Bible story of Nathanael, where Jesus told him he saw him under the tree long before either of them had met.

I have always loved nature and the outdoors and have felt there is a spiritual interconnectedness of nature and God's creatures. In my observation of the family farm and its seasonal operation, it seems to represent a perfect paradigm of a synergistic partnership with God.

As I reminisce on this topic, I recall that in the morning and evening my grandparents would gather the 25 dairy cows in the barn for "milking." Originally, they milked by hand, but by the time I arrived, they used milk machines. The other animals like the horses, pigs, and chickens also had to be fed. My grandmother had to collect the eggs, prepare the meals three times a day, clean the two-story brick house, and, if time allowed, work in her large garden or her flower yard. My grandfather would work the fields with his tractor, which was eventually replaced by a team of two large horses. He would mow the hay, plant the oats, and cultivate the corn. Sometimes we would fix the fences and repair the machinery. All was dependent on God for good weather and our prayer for an abundant harvest.

One of my favorite parts of each week was when we would take the pickup into town for groceries and go to the mill to grind our corn or oats for animal feed. Besides picking up groceries or going to the freezer for meat, my grandfather would always stop for a beer at the "beer joint" to visit with other farmers and share news. My brother and I would get a comic book to read while we patiently waited for him in the truck.

In those days, pet animals like Shep, our cattle dog, and the barn cats received little veterinary care. The feral cat population dwindled due to infectious disease and parasites, since they received no vaccinations. There was no spaying or neutering, either. We always had lots of kittens in the barn eating the left-over milk.

Shep loved to kill the snakes when they were uncovered by mowing the alfalfa field. One day, I remember accidently cutting Shep's leg while mowing hay and I think my grandfather took him in the woods and shot him. Those were the days of large animal veterinary practice (now called food animal practice). Small animal or pet practice was just beginning in the cities and in vet schools.

At that time, I observed my grandfather and his relationship with the farm veterinarian. The vet would come to our farm, periodically with his mobile hospital and care for all the cattle, horses, and pigs which were an important part of the operation. I noted that he was highly respected by my grandfather and others. So, I thought that would be a career to pursue someday. When asked the frequent question about my ambition at that time in my life, I started responding, "I'm going to be a vet!" To my satisfaction, that response seemed to please everyone.

As I look back to that time in my life, I see how things have changed in the past 50 years. The small family farms have all disappeared and we now have large acreage farms with advanced milking and crop operations. There are few veterinarians doing farm calls like there were in my grandparents' days.

Several years ago, when I was on the Florida Vet school admissions committee, interviewing potential vet school candidates, most of the candidates were women from urban backgrounds who were going into the occupation because of their love for small animals. My classes in vet school were men, mostly from farm backgrounds. We had three women in our class and now the classes have more than 80% women. My best friend in vet school was a large animal veterinarian. He tells me that in food animal practice, as it is now called, you can hardly make a living these days. In the past, he made a good living as a specialist in dairy cattle practice. Now much of the work in large animal surgery and medicine is being done by non-vet animal husbandry graduates.

PART II
THE
COLLEGE YEARS

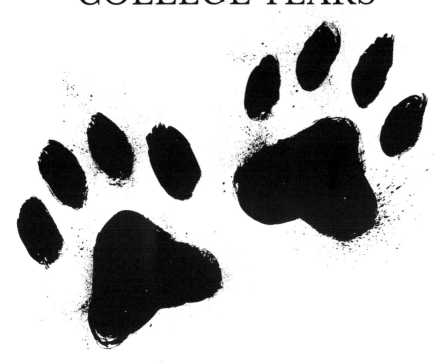

DR. BRUCE KEENE

CHAPTER 4

University of Arkansas: 1957-1961

UPON ARRIVING AT THE University of Arkansas for my freshman year at age 18, I still remember the apprehension I experienced the first night, away from home in a lonely motel room. I was thinking about the impossible road ahead. After all, I had spent most of my high school time in sports, avoiding the more difficult core courses required for pre-med like Algebra, Physics, and Chemistry. In fact, my freshman year at the University, I was so ill-prepared for college that I was required to take a non-credit English course to qualify for further coursework at the University of Arkansas.

In my desperation and lack of confidence, I said a prayer I've never forgotten. I promised God that if He'd help me get into vet school, I'd never forget Him doing that for me. I was certain that it was going to take a miracle.

My first semester at college I enrolled in the pre-med requisites - Physics and Organic Chemistry. However, I soon dropped out of both courses for fear of failure. I now know, after being on the vet school admissions committee, that those two courses are "make or break" requirements for all pre-vet students.

As mentioned prior, the courses for the vocation of veterinary medicine were all about farm animals. I was enrolled in Agriculture school, which was composed of primarily young men with farm backgrounds. Being from the city of Little Rock, Arkansas, I felt out of place being there. Although I studied hard, my classmates earned A's and I earned C's. I attributed that to their farm experience. Then, I found out they were studying from a fraternity library of old tests. From that time forward, my grades went up and I graduated with a B average. One of my proudest accomplishments in undergraduate school was taking Physics in summer school and getting a B without any high school math. Like I mentioned earlier, I have found that having good instinct makes all the difference in understanding a difficult subject.

CHAPTER 5

Kansas State University: 1961-1965

UPON GRADUATING WITH MY bachelor's degree in animal nutrition from the University of Arkansas, I was qualified for either graduate school in Nutrition or becoming a county agent. Neither of these were my first choice. At that point of my life, Vet school possibilities had become doubtful. There are only 27 veterinary schools in the US and there is a lot of competition. It has been said that it is easier to get into medical school than veterinary school. The State of Arkansas had an agreement with Oklahoma State to take three Arkansas applicants. However, there were many applicants better qualified than I for those slots. Once I had visited Oklahoma State Veterinary School, I became discouraged at my chances.

Also, upon graduation, my girlfriend at the time, Barbara, asked me to make a decision about our future. We decided to get married and I would go to graduate school in Nutrition. At that point, God started answering that prayer about school that I had made four years earlier, and He started engineering a miraculous series of events toward great opportunity. Because someone had told me that Kansas State University Veterinary School took a lot of out-of-state candidates, I sent my transcript to KSU and Dr. Lee Railsback, who was the Assistant Dean at that time. This helped my chances because Dr. Railsback had practiced in Arkansas before going to Kansas.

My fortune also turned because during the Cuban Missile Crisis, several students in the KSU freshman class had been drafted into service. This meant that three new students would be selected as replacements.

A day or so before my wedding day, I received a letter from Dr. Railsback inviting me to come for an interview. So, while on our honeymoon trip to Vicksburg, Mississippi, Barbara and I decided to turn around and drive 1000 miles northeast to Manhattan, Kansas.

After a successful interview, I was told that if I would take Physics in summer school and get a passing grade, I would be admitted to the freshman class. It was indeed a miracle!

We met classmates Randy Pederson and his wife Nancy from Nebraska that first year in 1961. Over the years, they have been our best friends. Since then, they have been like family to us. We lived as neighbors in the married student housing as we started our second year in Manhattan. At that time, they had a small daughter and Nancy also worked on campus.

During the four-year professional curriculum, I gradually realized that since I was from an urban background, I was more comfortable communicating with the small animal or pet clients. This was a fast-growing new area of opportunity in larger cities called companion animal practice. At KSU, we were fortunate to have a leader in this specialty. His name was Dr. Jake Mosher and he was also an excellent teacher. One other memorable small animal professor was Dr. Christianson. He was known by the students as an anal gland specialist. We shared a lot of special jokes in this regard!

DR. BRUCE KEENE

PART III
VETERINARY
PRACTICE WORK

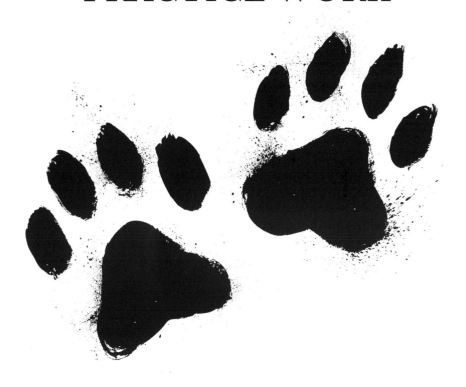

DR. BRUCE KEENE

CHAPTER 6

Magnolia, Arkansas Internship: 1964

DURING THE SUMMER BETWEEN my junior and senior year in vet school, I got a job with a mixed – small and large animals – practice in Magnolia, Arkansas. There were two Kansas State graduates in the practice, one older and one younger. The older had developed a contact allergy to blood and had to wear gloves all the time. At their hospital, they also had a kennel to board dogs and an apartment where I stayed. I could hear the dogs barking all night. There was an area for working on large animals in the back.

There are several memories I have of those summer experiences and I'd like to share a few.

Pet Skunks

One day a client brought in a litter of baby skunks that had been found orphaned by the mother who was killed by a car on the highway. This was common in that country area and you could smell them a mile away. The babies were less than a couple weeks old when I adopted the job of bottle feeding them every 3-4 hours. I was so much of their surrogate mother that they bonded with me and would follow me around everywhere I went. I have pictures to prove it. Evenings, I would lie on the apartment floor watching them play and they would romp around making their characteristic hard run ending with a tail up somersault. I knew this behavior was their defensive posture for spraying and I worried that would start while I was taking care of them. My plan was to de-scent them and sell them for a profit since they made popular pets at the time. They were so cute, and I became attached to them, even getting used to the odor. Looking back, I am amazed my bosses didn't kick us all out!

One day, I decided to try and de-scent a little male I had named Herman. You should understand, the only time I had witnessed this surgery before was when one of our professors in vet school had tried to de-scent a fully grown skunk. He protected himself against an accidental spraying by operating behind a window glass. However, he did accidently rupture the gland in surgery filling the area with a yellow putrid fume. That caused that portion of our small animal clinic to be shut down for several days.

To take care of Herman, I started by putting a cone over his nose to administer anesthesia. When he was asleep, I lifted his tail to look for the glands. Suddenly, a little pink nipple protruded out of the rectal area, pulsed, and skirted me right in the mouth. I ran to the bathroom and put my face in the shower head, washing my mouth. I assure you, it tastes worse than it smells. For those of you that have never smelled it, it must be like mustard gas in the military. I gathered myself and returned to the surgery site, this time placing a clamp on the gland duct. Then, I very carefully peeled out the small grape-like sacs. Later, I did become more confident doing that surgery and sold some of the skunks for $40 each. Skunks always attract quite a crowd of curious onlookers. Unfortunately, this was not the end of the story.

My wife, Barbara, became quite attached to one of the females named Priscilla. Priscilla, who loved crickets, accidently bit Barb's hand while she feeding her one day. One of the exotic animal disease facts I had not remembered from vet school was how highly susceptible skunks, raccoons, and bats are to the rabies virus. Back then, we had a dog and cat Modified Live Rabies vaccine that had enough potency to cause rabies in highly susceptible animals. Later, when Priscilla became paralyzed in her rear legs, I put two and two together and realized my vaccination had caused her to get rabies. Barbara tells how, when the lab report came back positive from the brain analysis for rabies, you could hear her scream all over the school she was teaching in. Since she had previously had the preventative series of shots from a childhood pet dog that had rabies, she only had to take a few additional boosters for protection. However, the shots are quite painful, and she's never forgotten my mistake.

A Sick Mule

One of my first cases as an intern involved a farm call with a sick mule. The scene was in an old shanty house owned by a black woman who was sitting on her front porch in her rocking chair. Across the porch were many empty bottles. These were left over from her previous attempts to use home remedies for the mules' colic, which is a belly ache caused by an obstruction of the intestines. I should mention that many of my early large animal patients would have already been treated by a local, non-graduate animal doctor or "quacks." In those days, graduate veterinarians were mostly not available. In fact, the Arkansas State Licensing Board would give you a license if you could prove you had made a living the last three years in "animal doctoring."

To help with my patient, I had a big strong, black man as my assistant from our clinic. He was skilled in large animal restraint, which is important working with cattle, horses, and mules. My patient was very weak, shaking, and in bad shape. My assistant put a twitch on her lip. A twitch is a device that when twisted causes some pain but diverts the mules' attention from kicking. That way, I could more safely examine and treat a horse or mule.

At that point of my understanding, I didn't know a blocked colon is usually hopeless without surgery. And this had to be done at a veterinary school hospital. Our standard treatment for most colic was a pain injection and passing a stomach tube down the horse or mules' nose into the stomach. This allowed me to pump a gallon of mineral oil down into the stomach to try to lubricate and break the blockage. Then you walk around with them so they do not lay down. Most milder cases would recover with this treatment. However, before I could get the tube passed on this mule, he shuddered and fell over dead. The old woman shook her head and said, "I guess I should have just given him another dose of Epson salts!" Obviously, she was not too impressed with the new vet.

The Preacher's Cow

On many of those first cases, like the mule, I felt I would have been better off to have been a preacher, so I could give the animal their last rites. In other words, they expected a miracle worker and as a vet, I was the last resort. Such was the case for an experience with one cow and a black preacher. I arrived late in the evening and to my frustration, he told me he didn't know where the animal was located in his large pasture. He told me the cow had been trying to deliver her calf for several days with no success. They had already tried to pull the calf out using a tractor and ropes connected to the calf legs with no success and by now the cow was in bad shape. We finally found her in a mud hole. The calf had been dead for some time, so my only hope would be to try to save the mother. This required an embryotomy which means removing the decaying, dead calf body in pieces. For over two hours, I labored in the blood and smelly afterbirth to remove all the body parts of the decomposed calf and finally, gave the mother supportive fluids and antibiotics. At the end, both my patient and I were not looking too good. Of course, I was not very optimistic for her recovery since she wasn't strong enough to even get up. Sure enough, she died during the night. Now as I look back, the humane thing to do would have been to call the rendering company and euthanize her.

Poor Judgement

One more learning experience I had during my internship was in the small animal or pet practice area. I had proudly diagnosed heartworm disease in one of our boarding dogs. These deadly parasites were common in South Arkansas. The parasites are spread by mosquitos and most dogs were kept outside the home because there were no leash laws in the town. Heartworms can grow to 12 inches long and live in the right chamber of the heart. They can multiply to as many as one hundred worms and kill a dog with heart failure by a year of age. When I diagnosed the parasites by seeing the little baby larvae under the microscope, I was excited to begin her treatment. This involved giving the dog four intravenous arsenic injections. Unfortunately, I proceeded with the treatment without talking to the owner. I just knew they would want her treated and applaud my cure when they returned. The problem was after the first injection the dog had a fatal reaction to the treatment and died in his cage. Of course, my poor judgement of not communicating the danger of treatment had been a disastrous mistake. There is always a danger in the treatment of this disease. Blood clots or pieces of the dying worms are infrequent but do occur. My employer had to take the responsibility for my action and buy the client a new dog.

Looking back now, I know it seems like I had a lot of failures. But after 50 plus years, I now know nothing can replace my experience as a teacher. I have never had a similar fatal heartworm treatment reaction since then and I went on to treat many dogs for heartworms in the years to follow. Also, after my large animal experiences, I am glad I didn't go into large animal practice.

CHAPTER 7

Dr. Yarborough, Miami: 1965

I PREVIOUSLY MENTIONED THAT during my senior year I took Dr Edwin Frick's advice to take a job in Miami, Florida. So, upon his recommendation my wife Barbara and I traveled from Manhattan, Kansas to Miami in 1965. I was 26 years old and recall my veterinary associate position was one of the best salaries offered at the time, raking in $1000/month.

My work in at Yarborough Animal Hospital consisted of working at one of three dog tracks each evening for 12 races and then being on emergency duty the rest of the night and working mornings 8:00 AM until noon with appointments at the hospital. Our professional staff, besides myself and Dr. Yarborough, included two married couples who were both veterinarians. One of them was Dr. Yarborough's son and daughter-in-law. He also had an older office manager named Marge, who kept the financial part of the practice fine-tuned. His plan of supplying young vets an excellent internship experience their first year and "picking their brains" for new information and cheap labor was a win-win situation for all of us.

At that time Dr. Yarborough had trained more vets in Florida than anyone else. He told me when he first came to Miami there were only three vet clinics in town. He was in his 80's and had suffered from polio in recent years requiring his kennel helper to get him out of bed each morning. He was a tough man and when he talked, everyone listened.

Yarborough Animal Hospital was a state-of-the-art, busy practice that cared for small animals only. In addition, his hospital included a large boarding facility in the heart of downtown Miami. As an example of how progressive his practice was, he even had a full-time vet technician. Once he sent me over to an equine hospital at the Hialeah horse racing track to give one of our surgery patients a post preventative radiation therapy.

Dr. Yarborough was also active in the community. He worked with the Miami Heart Institute in their research projects, and he helped greyhounds that were to be euthanized. The greyhounds also served as area blood donors for area veterinary clinics. He was also active in the Kiwanis Club, which is a community service group. This observation led me to later become a Rotary

Club member. I was able to get a lot of valuable experience and confidence that first year. However, one shortcoming of my experience there was that Dr. Yarborough only allowed his daughter-in-law and himself to perform all the surgeries.

During that year of working at the dog tracks my job was to check the dogs before each race and be available for emergencies. While sitting there for four hours each night, I made use of the time writing and publishing a manual of Dr Yarborough's expertise on his greyhounds, called *Lameness of the Racing Greyhound*. I took colored photos of our patients. A veterinary pharmaceutical company, named Upjohn, paid me a couple hundred dollars for my effort. The saddest part of working with the racing greyhounds was the large number of healthy, young dogs euthanized just because they were just not speedy enough. Since those early days, I am happy to report, we have several rescue groups seeking adoptions for these retired dogs and more people are aware of this tragedy. I have also continued rescue education projects and help supply greyhounds as blood donors rather than mere euthanasia.

Recently, the State of Florida voted to close its last dog tracks. I can understand this because in our state there are too many other ways to gamble. It has been a great memory for me to have had my experience with this unique breed of dogs. Their history dates to Kansas where they were used because of their 40 MPH speed to chase coyotes and jack rabbits for ranchers.

Later, when my wife and I interviewed Dr. Yarborough about his life story for our *Florida Vet Journal* article, I noticed that he had a Bible on his nightstand. I asked him if he had a personal faith. He said his favorite verse in the Bible was Proverbs 3:5-6, which has also been my favorite too. "Trust in the Lord with all thy heart and rely not on your own understanding and He will make your path straight." Dr. Yarborough was a great mentor for a young vet!

At that time, another pioneer leader and mentor for me in small animal medicine and surgery in Florida was Dr. Charlie Bild. He had also been a past employee of Dr. Yarbourgh. He was the founder of the American Animal Association, which has always been a premier benchmark for small animal practices in the United States. At one of our state meetings, Dr. Bild was moderator for what was called "Charlie's Quickies" – where veterinarians would share their practice tips. At one point, Charlie asked the audience if there were any new vets out there? I raised my hand and he tossed me a copy of *The Richest Man in Babylon*, a book of wisdom that helped me in my early years of practice. For instance, the book advised me to save one tenth of my income, no matter how much I made, and invest it well. It promised if I would do this, I would be assured of a good estate. This compounding principle has proven true for me in my 50 years of vet practice. One more favorite book of Charlie's was *Gretchen's Manual*, which was also filled with worldly wisdom for a young men and women.

At that time, passing the State Board in Florida was difficult, because, besides a written exam, the examining Board would give a practical exam. This part of the licensing was given at Dr. Clarence Dee's ranch. He was another pioneer in Florida vet med and one of Dr. Yarborough's friends. Actually, I think the exam was designed so that the Board could pass or fail anyone they wished. They wanted it to be that way because they thought there were just too many applicants who wanted a Florida license simply for their retirement years. After I took my practical test, which was a timed test, I knew I had not done well on the X-rays. For instance, one X-ray was of a child's foot to confuse you as with an equine patient's foot. I told Dr. Yarborough of my fear of failure and he advised me not to worry. He called Dr. Dee who agreed to let me come up to his farm again and take another look at the X-rays. However, Dr. Dee scared me when he proposed that he'd just let me spay a dog for him instead. With my inexperience in surgery, you can imagine my anxiety over that proposal. He was just pulling my leg though, and I passed. I believe these early vets set the tone for Florida's important role in national leadership in the industry to this day.

Soon after moving to Miami, my wife and I purchased a purebred Italian Greyhound named Tinkerbell as our first pet. If I had not been a veterinarian, we might have gone broke with her series of medical problems. She first had a broken front leg that took multiple surgeries. This was followed by mange, and then a broken tail.

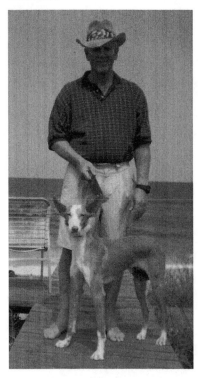

Our next hound breed was a Whippet named Isabelle. We loved all our dogs, but for me the dog that taught me the most about the human-animal bond was my Ibizan hound named Ibby. I had adopted Ibby as a 5-month-old Humane Society rescue operation. A breeder had abandoned a kennel of purebred Ibizan and there were three puppies up for adoption. I had always wanted this unique breed, but they were rare and awfully expensive. They originated from the Island of Ibiza, which is off the coast of Spain. They are the first cousin to the Pharaoh Hound pictured with the Egyptian pyramids. They are beautiful dogs built for speed and are like greyhounds, except that they have upright ears.

At first, Ibby was fearful because he had little social contact during his puppyhood. Soon after adopting him, we went on a beach walk where he pulled the retractable leash from my hand and with the handle chasing him, he escaped. With his 40 MPH speed he was quickly out of sight. I asked people on the sidewalk and highway next to the beach if they had seen him. One man told me he had jumped in a car with a good Samaritan. The man said if the owner showed up, he would have the dog at a location several miles closer to town. Thank God I got him back, but it took years for me to settle him down from his serious separation anxiety. He even chewed up my office door on one occasion. Over Ibby's 12-year life span, his unconditional love and devotion for me will always be a special memory.

On the outside of my veterinary practice life, Barbara and I lived in the suburb of Miami Springs, across the street from the Miami International Airport. All the neighbors in our apartment complex were either pilots or stewardesses. You can imagine the culture shock for two young naïve people from Arkansas adjusting to the fast-paced crowd in that environment.

While I was working my long hours, Barbara spent time at the pool getting a tan and making friends with our neighbors. One of those friends was a pilot that had taught flying in college, and he offered to teach her to fly. She started taking flying lessons in Miami and later completed her license in Orlando.

Our next-door neighbor was a stewardess named Janet. One day I had an opportunity to show off my experience in de-scenting skunks for her on a Florida spotted skunk, also known as a civet cat. These are different than the stripped variety of skunks I had raised in Arkansas. Janet volunteered to assist me. I told her I had been told that if you pick up a skunk by the tail, they will not spray you. She tried, but it didn't work, and he sprayed her!

Needless to say, she had to miss several flights the next week until the skunk odor disappeared. I found from that experience that the spotted skunk is much more difficult to de-scent. That was my first and last civet surgery. I would later try ferrets whom I also found to be difficult.

Next to our apartment was located the world-famous Miami Villas, a restaurant where many celebrities were seen. For instance, my wife saw TV personalities like Jackie Gleason, singer Frank Sinatra, and horse jockey Willie Shoemaker around our pool area while she was there. At our apartment that first year, there were many late-night, wild parties, and some of them were nude. It was an eye-opening experience for us.

Here is a list of a few of my most unusual patients that year:

The Anorexic Boa Constrictor

One day a client brought in a 10-foot-long boa constrictor that they said had not eaten for several weeks and was thin and emaciated. They told me his traditional meal was three rats every two weeks. You should know, I had no reptile course in vet school, so I was winging it with my treatment.

I instructed the client to bring me three rats. I first humanely euthanized the rats, which I now question, since the drug might have been poisonous for the snake too. Next, I had three helpers stretch the snake out full length and with forceps. I forced the intact rats through his mouth and worked them down to where I thought the stomach would be located. I was so proud of myself and I sent them home expecting good results. The next day the client called reporting the procedure had failed.

All three rats came out as feces without a hair being removed. In other words, no digestion!

I knew for other animals that are not eating, we often must force feed them by passing stomach tubes. I had also recently gone to the Miami Serpentarium and witnessed their venom collection and noted that they fed their snakes a liquid diet by stomach tube. So, that became my secondary plan. I had the client bring in three more rats but this time, I skinned them and placed the body parts in a blender and made a "rat milkshake." I then passed a stomach tube and this time it worked, and he recovered. You should have seen the expression on children's faces in elementary school volunteer programs when I tell that story. Gross!

Miss Honeysuckle White

It was Thanksgiving and grocery stores were selling lots of turkeys. One particular brand was advertised as having the most white meat. It was called Honeysuckle White. They had a mascot turkey visiting area grocery stores and her name was Miss Honeysuckle White. It was a hot Miami day and she came to our hospital with heat prostration. This problem is quite common in Florida with children and dogs being left in cars without ventilation. I jumped into our emergency routine for lowering animals high body temperature which is giving them a cold-water bath. A problem with avian species is that their normal body temperature is much higher than other species to begin with. It is about 105 degrees. Miss Honeysuckle White was panting uncomfortably. Fortunately, after our treatment, she regained consciousness and lived to continue her celebrity life.

Decrowing a Rooster

The final story involves a client that was requesting decrowing of their pet rooster. Their neighbors were up in arms about the 4:00 AM wakeup crowing and demanded something be done. In my notes from vet school there was a surgery described for debarking dogs by removing vocal cords. That is now considered inhumane. I also had some poultry notes on devocalizing roosters too, so I decided to give it a try. You should realize at this point in my career, I thought I had to learn how to do everything.

After putting the bird under gas anesthesia, I located the vocal cords near the chest. I clipped the two muscles that were recommended to devocalize birds. Later that day, I brought my patient out to the waiting room to meet the client, quite proud of my surgery. Suddenly, the rooster gave out the loudest crow you've ever heard. Naturally, I was as shocked as the client. All, I could do was apologize, and tell them there was obviously no charge and I never tried that again.

Crossett, Arkansas: 1967-1970

IN THE 10% OF my practice that was large animals like mules, horses, and cows, I had less experience and confidence. For instance, the first horse castration I was called to do, I was nervous. I had only castrated one testicle on one horse in vet school. I couldn't even find the jugular vein to administer the anesthesia. So, I used a front leg vein like I do in small animals. Somehow, I made it through that learning experience.

Anesthesia Accident

On another horse surgery, I had asked a young vet about his anesthesia technique and he told me he had a proven method. He used an anesthetic that had a dose of one vial per 250 pounds of body weight. So, I calculated for a 1000-pound horse, I would use four vials, and this would give me just enough time to get the job done. The horse dropped immediately as planned, but I noticed he wasn't breathing. I tried my best to give him artificial respiration, but without success. There are always dangers with giving anesthesia, but later I learned most anesthesia drugs are used "to effect" – which means as little as needed is used and never in a bolus as I had done. After that disaster, all I could do was to offer to buy the client another horse and I certainly learned an important lesson about being careful and taking all advice. Of course, I was sorry for my mistake.

Thankfully, I lived through all these tough learning experiences, and after three years had a thriving practice with a small number of large animal calls.

Maude and Zip-Zip

In my clinic, I had a three-legged Walker Hound named Maude. She had been given to me because she was gun shy. Also, she had lost her back leg by having it caught in a fence chasing deer. Since there was no leash law in town, I was able to let her run around the neighborhood behind my clinic. When I needed her for a blood transfusion, I simply went to the front door and called her. She saved many lives with her blood because hookworm disease was common in the area. I had also planned to breed her thinking raising a litter of puppies in a hunting area would be profitable. I was successful in raising a large litter of healthy pups, but because I had bred her at the wrong time of the year, I had to give all of them

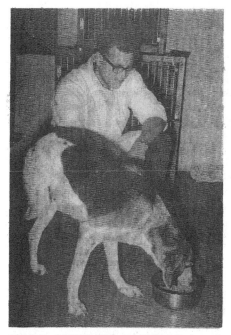

SPECIAL TREAT FOR MAUDE follows each blood-letting. Here the three-legged pet of the Crossett Animal Clinic ties into a very meaty meal while Dr. Keene looks on.

away for free because they were too costly to feed.

I also had a clinic mascot Siamese cat named Zip-Zip. She was best buddies with Maude. There was even a feature article written about the two of them in the state newspaper, *The Arkansas Gazette.* Everyone loved them because the two were always cuddled up together in my waiting room. One day, Zip-Zip disappeared. I thought someone must have stolen her. About six months later, a client told me they had seen her on a picnic table in the backyard of a house on the other side of town. I drove over, picked her up, and brought her back. I believe she must have crawled into the back seat of a client's car one day and found another family to take care of her.

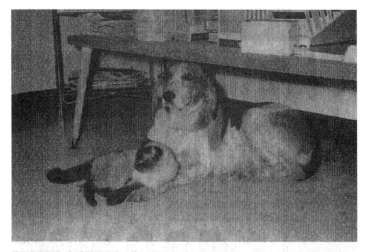

FOSTER SISTERS - People have become accustomed at the Crossett Animal Clinic to seeing Maude and Zip-Zip resting together under the low table in the Reception Room. While they are about as extremely opposite in appearance as two creatures can be and still bear fur, they do not seem to be aware of the fact that they are not of the same race, creed and color.

Mosquitos & Heartworms

Once, I had a client's dog whom I had treated for heartworms who had a reaction while I was attending a weekend vet meeting out of town. When I returned Monday morning, the client was waiting for me and was very angry. He verbally attacked me because I was gone and not there to treat his dog. He also didn't like that he had to go to another town to another vet for extra treatment for the reaction. This was a short man and he put his finger in my chest and proclaimed, "From now on you're Mr. to me!" I was getting angry myself by then and was trying to think about what to do. My reception-ist, Marge, was begging me not to hit him. So, I lifted him up and tossed him to the floor pinning him there trying to get him to cool down and give me time to think about what to do. I decided it was my office and I didn't have to put up with that verbal abuse, so I tossed him out the front door of the clinic. Of course, I started worrying about how this event would play out in the community. I thought I might get a bad reputation that would ruin my great start in my first practice. You must understand that I'm usually a quiet, peace-loving man with no anger problem. However, the story does have a happy ending because this man was known for his tem-per and similar behavior in the past and later admit-ted he got what he deserved. I still have a cartoon that was posted humorously on the town paper mill bulletin board depicting the event.

Hog lice and a C-section

One of my first patients was a 200-pound female hog who was pregnant and having a difficult delivery. Again, with little farm animal experience to rely on, I went to my small animal experience and took her into my surgery room and operating table. I gave her anes-thesia and with my wife's assistance preceded to do a C-section. This is a mid-line abdominal incision and by cutting into the uterus or birth canal, I removed eight cute little baby pigs. My wife's job was to briskly rub the babies, clean their nostrils of mucus and make sure they squealed with new life. She did a good job. She will never forget the experience.

The surgery room floor was one inch thick with fatty fluid. The excessive fat on pigs makes a C-section on a pig much different than one performed on a dog. On top of that, the mother pig was loaded with lice. The lice got on everything! I was glad the family went home with the mother and babies doing well and that I never again had to do a pig C-section or delivery.

Bulldog C-section and Sugar Bowl

Another patient I will never forget was an English bulldog. She was very spoiled. For example, when we boarded her, we had to go to Dairy Queen daily for her ice cream cone. English bulldogs are known for their difficult pregnancies and I would later learn almost all of them require a C-section like the previous pig patient. The mother's delivery date is usually about 63 days after gestation and was close to New Year's Day at the time. I was scheduled to go to a Sugar Bowl game for my Alma Mater, Arkansas Razorbacks football game that weekend. As you probably guessed, my patient started her delivery the night before my trip. Her delivery was slow, having about two pups every hour. Often, I'd have to assist her with injections to increase her contractions or physically having to help pull them out of the birth canal. The last puppy of her eight-baby litter wouldn't budge. So, I had to miss my bowl game and perform a C-section for one pup. If that was not frustrating enough, the same dog repeated a second difficult delivery the following year resulting in another C-section for the last pup. I swore after that, to always recommend C-sections for that breed. Memories like this make me thankful for that later in my practice I started an after-hours emergency veterinary center.

My Invention

You will recall from my vet school experience with Dr. Christianson, I became good at removing anal sacs in dogs, cats, and skunks. Most vets are probably afraid of doing this surgery because one complication after surgery can be the loss of bowel function if the rectal sphincter is damaged. The other problem of this surgical procedure is that it requires an assistant help hold multiple forceps. I decided I would develop an instrument (a medical surgery retractor) allowing me to do the surgery without help. It was a circular ring with six clamps around the outside. I had a local machine shop develop my prototype instrument. I even published an article in a vet journal showing the procedure and demonstrated the use at a local vet meeting. However, because of the low number of veterinarians doing this operation and the high cost of patenting, I had to abandon the effort.

Big Game Hunter

Another idea I had in Crossett was to become a big game hunter. Our area was all about outdoor living, fishing, and deer hunting. I had watched on television the African safari where they used capture guns to immobilize various wild animals. We had some experiences in vet school with the local zoo. So, I purchased a capture rifle of my own. I thought it would be good to have one for my cattle patients and maybe deer hunting. This turned out to be very frustrating because I found to load the syringes was quite expensive. Also, my early shooting resulted in many misses and lost syringes. I decided to rent the rifle to clients rather than use it myself. The other thing was most of the quick knock down drugs were dangerous and were slow to take effect. This required tracking the animal long distances after being shot and I was not interested in doing that.

A Miracle

Horses can be dangerous for a veterinarian to work on and the owners also can be difficult to work with. One horse and his owner fit both of these descriptions. I decided to use a drug, which was a controversial muscle paralysis compound that required local anesthesia for pain control. It was not unlike the curare in African native blow guns. After my earlier anesthesia accident on the horse castration, you can imagine my nervousness about equine anesthesia. This horse needed to have a cancerous growth taken off his back leg and I knew he was very skeptical of my young vet abilities. I knew with this drug I would have to work quickly. All went well and just as I finished and bandaged the leg, the horse jumped to his feet, shook and walked away. The man stood there in amazement as if I had just performed a miracle. I was thankful, but never tried that method again.

The Rodeo Bull

One last case I recall was being asked to treat a rodeo bull in town for our annual rodeo event. My only memory of bulls was when I almost signed up to ride one at college. Fear and better judgement prevailed at that time. I was pretty scared this time, too. This bull had an injured penis. The cowboys loaded him into the chute allowing me to inject a tranquilizer into his tail vein. He laid down in the bottom of the chute and they opened it where I could clean and treat the wound. My treatment came out surprising well that time too.

Old South Lesson

I practiced in Crossett for three years and the residents were really good to me. However, I decided I was too isolated and would have more opportunity for professional growth and continuing education in a bigger place. So, I decided to go back to Florida with a classmate who was also practicing in Arkansas. I had previously found him a job working with me in Miami. I advertised to sell my practice and had two vets interested. One was a white man from a town not far away. The other man was a black graduate from Tuskegee Veterinary School. Since I was looking for the best qualified, I chose the black vet. I had no idea of the remaining racial prejudice in my area until one of my favorite "redneck character" clients came in and angrily complained that I had done the community a disservice by choosing a "nigger."

PART IV
JOINING FORCES
IN VETERINARY
MEDICINE

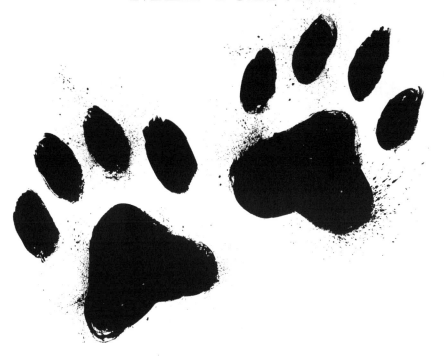

DR. BRUCE KEENE

CHAPTER 9

Howell Branch Animal Hospital: 1970

A KANSAS STATE CLASSMATE and I had stayed in touch, both practicing first in Florida, then Arkansas. We decided to form a partnership and move back to Florida. We felt there would be more opportunity for our future there. We also knew that Orlando, Florida was going to be a "boom town" with the announcement that Disney World was coming to the Central Florida area in two years. After a lot of searching and taking advantage of a rare zoning opportunity, I found a strategically located property in the community of Winter Park, Florida which is a suburb of Orlando. This gave us our God-given opportunity. Finding land zoned for a veterinary clinic in a residential area is very difficult. The front building on our property had been most recently a fruit stand. When we first started Howell Branch Animal Hospital in 1970, our vet practice was in a converted home and people passing by on the busy frontage road would see us doing surgery in the living room. They probably couldn't believe their eyes!

We built our practice rapidly by taking emergency night calls and doing large animal practice, mostly horses. There were few local veterinarians interested in these "country calls." As we had hoped, in just three years, we added a third vet to practice exclusively for large animal work. We also built a state-of-the-art small animal hospital on our property.

The local vet association had rotating emergency duty at that time which we did not join initially because we needed the emergency income. The local association was upset with us for this decision. I'll never forget that I was even called before the local association board to defend our ethics. They accused us of stealing other clinics' clients because we were in competition with their emergency services. The problem was that the others in our area required clients to travel miles for their "on call" emergency clinic and we were closer and more available when they were closed.

Ironically, after my first bad experience with the veterinary association in the area, I put together a co-op group of 15 investor clinics that would form the

Veterinary Emergency Clinic of Central Florida. My wife found the property while antique shopping, and it was a local crematory. This successful partnership of 15 original investors has since grown to over a hundred clinics in four locations in Central Florida. During our first years, the member clinics would rotate night duty for one weekend and one weeknight, but now we have full-time staff veterinarians. It is one of my proudest accomplishments.

DR. BRUCE KEENE

CHAPTER 10

Stories from my Veterinary Clinic

A Fishy Tale/Dr. Dog

My neighborhood medical doctor friend, Bill, invited me to play poker with his doctor friends who had also retired from our local naval base. They would always have a good laugh over my emergency calls. Once, a client called me about her sick fish. I had no idea from the symptoms what was wrong since that was not a part of my veterinary education. So, I called one of my clients who had a hobby raising fish. She told me after describing the sick fish symptoms, to "flush it." I guess the contagious aspects and concern for the other fish didn't allow individual treatment. This is much like the livestock industry where herd health is the concern. It was in this group of friends where I was first called Dr. Dog.

African Party

One of our poker playing buddies was a pawn shop owner. He had evidently been quite financially successful in his business. He had a girlfriend who had a love for animals, and he supported her passion. In fact, at their estate home, they had a collection of exotic cats which included a cougar, leopard, and a panther. He also bought her a pet shop business. I took care of their animals. In those days, my wife and her friend gave an African Party as one of their themed parties. I supplied animals from the pet shop. I had a beautiful scarlet macaw at the front door to welcome the guests. In our master bedroom, I had an ocelot, which is a small exotic cat the size of a bobcat. He would hide under our bed and when the guests would go into the bathroom, he would charge them and playfully grab their leg. As you can imagine, that was quite exciting. No liability issues came up though – thank God!

A Bear Story

In the front window of the pet shop, they had a Malayan Sun Bear for sale. This is a beautiful black bear from Indonesia that has a large white star on its chest. They weigh about 150 pounds and stand about 5 feet tall. One night, I received an emergency call from a young couple who had purchased that bear. They lived in an apartment close to our clinic and the bear had gone crazy in the confinement of their small apartment. He was tearing the carpet off the floor and taking large sections out of the drywall. The apartment manager was threatening them with eviction. This bear was friendly, but strong.

I sent our cowboy veterinary helper, whom we used for our large animal calls to handle dangerous cattle and horses. I sent a couple injections of tranquilizer and a stainless-steel cage with him. About an hour later, he called reporting that he had no success getting the bear into the cage. This time, I sent stronger drugs and finally, after another hour of struggle, the bear was loaded and on his way to our clinic. By the time he arrived, he was waking up and tearing the door off our stainless-steel cage. Hurriedly, we remodeled the old house in the back of our clinic for his confinement. He was so strong, his claws were digging through concrete block walls.

For a while, we had fun showing him to clients and visitors. One evening I brought my medical doctor neighbor Bill to see him and told him the bear loved to have his chin scratched. He crawled into the pen and then I told him that he was the first person to have done that. He turned pale white and got out of the pen quickly, not appreciating my practical joke at all. Actually, I knew it was safe.

Another time, I decided I would put a collar on the bear so I could take him places on a leash. He would have nothing to do with my plan. He gave me a look like "you've got to be kidding." His favorite treat was a large can of Hawaiian Punch. He'd rip the top of can off and chug it. This caused quite a case of diarrhea.

Finally, when a local newspaper ran an article about him, a wildlife park in North Carolina offered to take him and give him a good home. We were more than ready to agree to that offer.

The Pet Fair

Soon after starting practice in Orlando, I was asked to be a judge at an annual Pet Fair, which was the major fundraising event for the Orlando Science Center (OSC). The OSC is a hands-on teaching museum that features a large telescope and planetarium. The Pet Fair was a winter carnival with fun pet judging for mostly children's pets in various categories ranging from "best dressed" to "best trick" or "best in breed" like sporting or toy. In the beginning, I also judged snakes, cats, birds, and even one little girl brought a quail she had hatched and raised. Also, one contestant had a tarantula and another, Madagascar cockroaches. One year, a lady brought a horse in a trailer, but we had to explain to her the contest was only for small pets.

I always thought the Orlando Science Center would be an excellent opportunity for client education in veterinary medicine and surgery. On several occasions, I carried my surgery table to the facility and performed live spay and castration operations. I also invited my colleagues to demonstrate sexing birds. And even once we had a cataract surgery demonstrated by a veterinary ophthalmologist friend. Later, I got our local vet group involved and we performed mini physical exams and referred them to their local vets if needed. We also involved veterinary pharmaceutical and pet food corporate sponsors, which raised a lot of money for the center.

Rotary Pig

From my time in Miami with Dr. Yarborough's mentoring, I learned to be involved with volunteerism through membership in civic service groups. In Crossett, I was a Jaycee and in Orlando, I became a Rotarian. My club was a breakfast club and the diversity of the vocations and friendships I developed in those 20 plus years is a wonderful memory. One of our morning activities was the practice of having "bragging bucks." This was where you place a dollar in the piggy bank, and you got to brag about anything you were proud of the past week. This had replaced the old practice of fining people for being late or carrying a teddy bear for a week. That almost caused me to resign in the beginning! Being a graduate of the University of Arkansas, whose mascot is a pig or Razorback, every time my team would win a game, I'd pay a buck and have the club give a loud "Wooo-pig sooie!" This is the team's famous cheerleading yell. Actually, my Rotary club got better at calling the hogs than the native Arkansans over the years.

Periodically, I would have the monthly club responsibility of providing the morning program. Since my classification was vet med, naturally Dr. Dog chose an animal related topic. I decided to invite the local Humane Society and since they had a potbellied pig up for adoption, I asked them to bring him along. My plan was to pull a practical joke on my club members and when they gave a hog call that morning, I told my Humane Society guests to let the pig run into the breakfast hall. I was going to tell my fellow Rotarians that they had become so good at calling the hogs, that the Florida wild hogs were coming in from the surrounding woods. Now, I have been told pigs are very intelligent and what happened next makes me think that's true. The joke completely backfired on me. This little pig ran right over to my chair out of the 30 people he could have selected and made a mess. And of course, I had to clean it up.

DR. BRUCE KEENE

CHAPTER 11

Lake Howell Animal Hospital - Deltona: 1976-2006

AFTER FOUR YEARS, MY partnership was beginning to have problems with my partner having affairs, a divorce, and with us discovering we had different practice philosophies. I decided I was happiest with a smaller "mom and pop" practice. I preferred a slower pace with a client-oriented practice. My partner wanted to have a bigger practice, make lots of money, and grow. I call that stressful time in our life, the "Rise and Fall of the Roman Empire." At the end, I could see a long, bitter, legal battle with only the attorneys coming out on top. During that stressful year, for the first time in my life, I even started taking tranquilizers, which I said I'd never do. Without the help of my faith, and a good

Christian attorney friend, I don't know what I would have done. The final agreement involved me leaving the practice and starting over with my partner assuming quite a lot of past debt, but a good location and a clinic with a good clientele. I did not get much equity for six years of hard work, but was able to purchase a home and acreage nearby to start over. Unfortunately for me, since we had trained our clients to see either of us over the years, my partner retained most of our clients.

A Swimming Pool Miracle

What happened next is another example of God's engineering my life for His purpose. I was sitting in my home office contemplating my future when one of the miracles in my life occurred. First, please understand. I would not have been at home that day if I had not been out of work.

I remember hearing a scream from our backyard pool area and my daughter came to my office reporting that Bryce, our two-year-old son was dead. My wife was in shock and no one knew CPR. When I rushed to our backyard pool, our six-year-old daughter, a strong swimmer, had pulled our son off the bottom of the pool. By the time I got to the pool deck, my son was blue, not breathing and there was no sign of life. Our maid, Ella, who had been more of a surrogate mother to our children since my wife and I both worked out of the home, was on the back porch wringing her hands and praying to Jesus. I picked my son up by his feet and shook him and water poured out his mouth and nose. I first tried artificial respiration, but had no confidence in it and I had no results, so I took him over to the lawn area and did the old fashioned resuscitation method I had been taught from my YMCA life guarding days. I was the only one at home that day that knew CPR. The thought racing through my mind at that time was the fear that we were going to have a dead or brain damaged child. Pool accidents are all too common in Florida.

I knew in my experiences with animal resuscitation, the odds are against you. I also thought of the story of the bird in the young man's hand. When asked if the bird were alive or dead, the wise old man knew the boy was trying to trick him and told him "the answer is up to you." That day God answered Ella's and my prayers and gave my son life. The time to prevent brain damage or death in these swimming pool accidents is minutes. The emergency call response was over 30 minutes because we were outside the emergency zone. Later, we took him to the hospital where an X-ray showed enlarged heart from water intake, but no other problems. Praise God!

So, for the second time in Orlando, I was starting a new practice. I made a vow this time that my new partnership would be with the Lord and he would have 51% interest. At that time, my church and friends supported me in the transitional facility I was working on. The two acres I purchased was on a major intersection from a hard-nosed older man who told me the property was $75,000, "take it or leave it and next year it'll be more." He also said it would take several months to move out, giving me a dirty garage to practice out of in the transition. I did my best to create a surgery and exam area with a small back room as my cage area.

Deltona Satellite

To get extra clients, I also started a practice in Deltona, Florida which at the time, had no vet. I would commute from my location during the noon hours for afternoon office hours there. I drove 30 minutes daily to the northern suburb of Orlando called Deltona. While there, I would have a couple hours of appointments in a shopping center lease office and transport my surgery patients back in my car to Orlando. In both locations, I had gone back to the smaller, more personal practice that I had left in Crossett. During the half hour commute, I made use of my travel time by reading the entire Bible for the first time in my life. I had a Tornado Oldsmobile, which I considered very safe on the highway and traffic was light then on I4. A little old lady at church reminded me one time "don't you know the Bible is on tape?"

Between the two practices, I grew quickly, and after two years, sold my shopping center practice and a future building site next door. I realized without moving there and building a new vet facility, the competition would arrive soon.

Back at Lake Howell

At Lake Howell, we had office prayer each morning and I was blessed to have an older man and groomer named Jim Brown as my Christian mentor who was experienced and supportive of me. This was important for my staff's harmony. As an example, one of my receptionists, who later committed suicide, had once told her friend that our clinic's prayer time was especially important to her during an abusive marriage relationship.

Another important mentor I had following a Christian retreat I attended called "Cursillo" was Frank Temple. He was an older insurance agent who really loved our Lord. I had a men's group with him once a week and his favorite daily devotional was from Oswald Chambers. It was called *My Utmost for His Highest*, which I have continued to read every day since.

At Lake Howell, after I was able to move into the entire house, things started getting better. I remodeled it into a very workable clinic and even had an apartment in the back for my mother and father-in-law when they moved to Orlando. After 10 years, I built Keene Kennel where I could board 50 dogs and 20 cats.

For thirty years from 1976-2006, I practiced veterinary medicine and surgery at Lake Howell Animal Hospital. I would like to share with you some of my favorite memories of that time.

PART V
FINAL STORIES

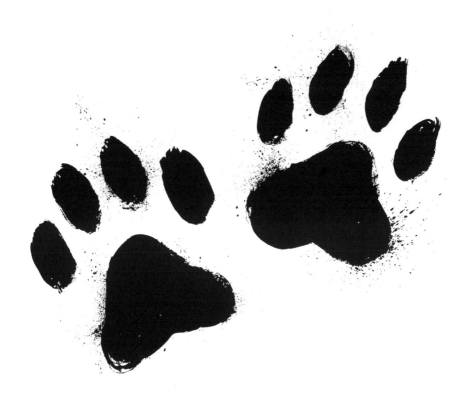

CHAPTER 12

Entertaining Tales from my Life as a Vet at Lake Howell Animal Hospital

Sarah, my talking parrot

Soon after opening my practice, I decided there was an opportunity to specialize in pet birds or avian medicine and surgery. I was taking care of a pet shop close to my clinic and so, without any vet school education, except in poultry, I had to learn quickly how to care for birds. I started by buying books, studying everything available on birds, and going to continuing education courses. Because one of my clients was a "character named Boyd" who was custodian of our local hotel zoo, I also needed to learn how to surgically determine the sex of his birds along with taking care of his 10-foot-long boa constrictor. I decided to purchase my first parrot as a learning project. I had been given many abandoned love birds, parakeets, and cockatiels by clients, but none of the larger avian varieties like the macaws, cockatoos or parrots to treat.

One of my clients imported parrots through Miami and I asked him to get me an African Grey Parrot. They are said to be the best talkers of all birds. I named my parrot, Sarah. She was six months old when I bought her for $500. She was a beautiful grey color with bright red tail feathers. I had a wooden perch constructed in our waiting room and Sarah would sit there, unattended, entertaining the waiting room clients, but had not started talking yet. Someone had told me the best method to teach a bird to talk was to make a continuous tape recording of what you want them to say and then play it repetitively to them. I was determined not to have a dirty talking parrot, like those I had heard of, so I had one young lady record "Praise the Lord" over and over for me. I thought Sarah could be my "Christian witness," since my wife told me I could not display my wooden cross in the waiting room. She thought that would offend my Jewish clients. After several months playing that recording, I gave up on Sarah learning anything and decided I just had a "dumb" parrot. Then one day, a drug rep was sitting in the waiting room next to Sarah's perch when she blurted out "Praise the Lord."

The salesman just about fell out of his chair. He later asked my Christian receptionist if she was "born again." After that, Sarah 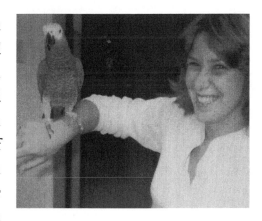 started mimicking all kinds of different peoples' voices, quail calls from outside the clinic, and even the telephone ringing.

I thought one day I had lost her because I had failed to clip the wing feathers on one side to prevent her from flying. She flew off her perch into the ceiling fan and was "knocked out" cold. I rushed her to my surgery room and after giving her oxygen she regained consciousness. It was a "praise the Lord" moment indeed! She did have seizures for a while after that from her concussion but had no long-term effects.

Sarah was a picky eater and ate mostly sunflower seeds that probably led to some poor health. Finally, she developed liver problems and I lost her after only a few years. I did have a lot of fun with her and took her with me on many of my school visits. Usually, parrots live as long as humans, but they can pick up infections from people, like those in my waiting room, which I assumed was the case.

A cat named Boodles

I had other pets in my clinic during my thirty years at Lake Howell. One of my favorites was a black, long-haired cat named Boodles. He was the pet of a man and woman who were artists and traveled a lot to art shows all over the country. Boodles became my star boarder. When he got older, he lost his sight and the clients were going to put him to sleep. We were all so used to giving him full use of the clinic that we offered him a permanent home. Even without his sight, he got around the clinic without bumping into anything.

Billy

I also had a large, black and white cat named Billy. Whenever anyone would go into our bathroom, he would run in there with them and compulsively start eating. He undermined my credibility with my clients of preaching dieting for pets as he became quite obese. When I retired, one of my old clients asked to adopt Billy and little did I know I had at one time given them Billy's sister.

Beau and Toes

I also had two retired racing greyhounds that were kept in my kennel as resident blood donors. They were what greyhound people called "easy keepers." They were very loving and friendly. One was Beau and the other was Toes. While working with the greyhounds, I also found blood donors for several other area clinics. After my experience in Miami, I thought I could specialize in working with these fine athletes, but found the industry was difficult to work for because trainers did most of their own vet work. It reminded me of my practice in Arkansas. There, they only relied on vets for the tough problems that they had failed to fix. Also, it is a sad industry because, as you recall from my Miami days, only the best greyhounds are eligible to receive treatment and surgery. By the time a racing dog gets to the track, the owner has likely invested thousands into their training. In my later years, I have become their advocate by taking a wonderful, greyhound dog named "Doc" to schools to encourage adoptions. I work with an older couple that has dedicated their retirement years to finding homes and boarding greyhounds while families are away. Over my lifetime, great success has been accomplished toward educating the public about the tragedy of the breed's genocide.

The Prosecuting Attorney

I have always been active in my church since starting my practice in Orlando. In fact, my church supporters and friends were important in starting over at Lake Howell. Soon after my new beginning, I went on a weekend Christian retreat with a group of men from our Diocese. One of the leaders of the team was a prosecuting attorney for the City of Orlando. During that weekend of fellowship and teaching, the attorney and I became friends. He called me the following Monday morning after I returned. It seemed their family pet, a small dog that was his son's best friend, had developed heartworm disease. With great concern, they decided they would trust me to treat him. The next morning, they brought the nervous Chihuahua into the clinic. A member of my staff put the dog in a cage near the surgery room. Unfortunately, they failed to latch the cage door securely and he jumped to the floor, running out of the front door of my clinic just as a client was entering. The fast, frightened, little dog ran across my big front yard into the busy traffic in front of my clinic and in an instant was struck by a car and killed.

Of course, when I learned about this tragic accident, I knew I was responsible and could only imagine the worst possible outcome. Malpractice is not a big problem in veterinary medicine, but a prosecuting attorney's dog? I prayed, *"Well Lord, now we'll see how this Christian forgiveness really works."* I called my friend and truthfully explained the details and after a long silence he simply said, "I'll get back to you." I remember thinking, *"I'll bet you will a big lawsuit."* A few days later, I had a call from the lawyer's oldest son. He said, "Dr. Keene, I want you to know, I forgive you." How important was that event for teaching a child a lesson in forgiveness!

Role Reversal

One day, a client brought me an unusual case involving a two-foot-long, red-tailed python. It seems the snake had become the victim, rather than the predator, for a small, white rat that was to be his meal. The snake had been bitten on his tail by the rat after the rat became bored with the python's lack of interest in him. Gangrene or death of tissue had occurred in the tail and it would require amputation. I questioned what I could use for anesthesia as you know from my story of the anorexic Miami Boa, I had little reptile experience. I did know that a snake's metabolism slows down in cold weather and they go into a dormant, hibernation stage of living. So, I put the snake in my freezer for a period necessary to force a "sleep" or provide a crude form of hypothermia anesthesia. I performed my surgery successfully and then warmed him up back to room temperature. Since that time, I learned a much better method of anesthesia from a veterinarian and exotic specialist at my old practice. I recently watched him conduct a C-section on an egg-bound corn snake. His anesthesia method was just like we use on dogs, cats, and horses. He placed a tracheal tube in their airway and gave the snake an anesthesia gas. During the surgery you could listen to the snake's breathing and heart rate just like any other species of animal.

Pampered Pets

In my practice area of Winter Park, Florida, there have always been many wealthy northerners who have maintained large winter homes. Hugh McCain owned much of the land in our area and had a mansion and beautiful lakeside estate grounds. He shared the park drive with the public by allowing a road through their property. He also had a flock of peacocks along the drive for people to enjoy watching. He was a big benefactor for the city, providing the community an art museum of his Tiffany glass art collection. And he was a client of mine.

Mr. McCain employed a retired sheriff of the city, Carl Buchanan, as his personal bodyguard and chauffeur. This person was tasked with bringing the family's beloved, Holly, a cocker spaniel, to me for vet work. On one occasion, the millionaire made a personal appearance by bringing an albino, baby peacock in for me to treat. I will never forget seeing this rich and famous man, lying on my surgery floor with that little bird running all over his chest. I thought at the time of how the love of animals brings people to a common place of compassion without regard for worldly status.

Still another client of mine was a wealthy couple who were very active in supporting the arts in our area. They also lived in a beautiful mansion on a lake near our home. I took care of their Yorkshire terrier named Gucci, who was a geriatric patient living well past everyone's expectations. I also cared for their parrot, Malcolm. Because I was their vet, I was always invited to their annual Christmas party that was attended by only a select few in the area - mostly politicians and dignitaries. I would joke with a tennis friend, who was a county commissioner, whether he had received an invitation or not like I had.

On one occasion, the lady of the house asked me to come over to trim Malcolm's toenails. I asked her to hold him wrapped in a towel. Besides their sharp toenails, their strong beaks can break a finger. About halfway through the procedure, she panicked when Malcolm struggled and she let him go. He went right for her hand. Thank God she was wearing the biggest diamond ring you have ever seen, and he bit it! Parrots are attracted to bright objects. Another "praise the Lord" moment!

The Stripper

I will never forget the client who was a provocatively dressed woman with the perfect body. She was a body builder stripper who used her assets and a lot of plastic surgery to practice her trade. She worked only in the highest quality clubs in Florida. Her two dogs were chow-chows, a black one and a white one. One day, the black one was brought to me because he was lame. I had her bring the two dogs into my backyard to observe the lameness and immediately they got into a big fight. There was black and white fur flying everywhere when suddenly the stripper, without worrying about her own safety, got in between them and broke it up. I commented, "I'll bet you don't have much trouble with men making passes at you?" She said, "No, but I've had to knock over a few off bar stools."

After treating her dogs, she asked me if I had any anabolic steroids and I got a clearer understanding of how she built that body of muscles. When I started in greyhound practice, the trainers used these drugs as the human athletes do to get an advantage in bodybuilding. Over the years, I have been aware of several drugs that have been the subject of misuse by humans and required careful security control.

A Grooming Tragedy

A cat incident I'll never forget involved a long-time client that left his cat with me for a bath. I was in surgery when I heard screaming from the bathing area and it appeared the groomer had tied the cat to the tub grill in such a way the cat had jumped off the table and hung herself. The vet tech had discovered the groomer's negligence and they were about to get into a fight when I arrived. I tried to resuscitate the cat without success. The angry tech called the police, who contacted the news media. I called my client and again explained the accident truthfully. They accepted my explanation because of our long and trusted relationship. They even dismissed any cooperation for a media story of neglect which protected my hospital's reputation. I think this is a good example of client loyalty which I am so thankful for during those 30 years at Lake Howell.

The Deacon and Barnie

One of my favorite patients was an older hound named Barnie. He was the grand dog of our deacon who lived in a home next to our church. The deacon often joked about our Arkansas roots with my mother-in-law who lived in the back of my clinic. He said I was Barnie's godfather. Every morning Barnie, with his old age, required the deacon to get up for his bathroom break.

One time, I had to treat a hot spot, which is a self-inflicted skin sore that required an Elizabethan collar to be placed around the neck to protect the pet from reaching the area. The deacon told me on the way out from my clinic that he had to take the collar off because he was embarrassed by people's stares seeing both of them wearing collars.

Immigration and an Animal Rights Attorney

One female client I had was a very distinguished attorney. She held a PhD from the University of Illinois. Dr. Dunbar was proud of the fact that she was the first female attorney to argue a case before the Supreme Court of Illinois. One of her best friends was the Dean of the School of Veterinary Medicine at the University of Illinois. As a single woman, her family was made up of several adopted dogs.

She was one of my most unusual and demanding clients I have ever had. She required a lot of special attention. I provided house calls on several occasions. She once told me the way she adopted pets was to ask for the most un-adoptable dog in the shelter. Whenever I treated a difficult case, I always had to consult with the Dean of the Veterinary School in Illinois or Florida for confirmation of my treatment. Once a year in her home she held a neighborhood champagne reception in memory of any animal friends lost by her guests. Some of her friends stayed in touch through long distance telephone calls.

In her college days, she had taught an animal law course and since retiring, she has sponsored animal law courses at several law schools across the country. She was also a regular speaker on animal law at many veterinary schools. She was quite wealthy and has provided an animal chapel for her alma mater.

One day, she came to me with a strange request. She asked me if I would be the veterinary job site for young woman from the University of Illinois whom she was seeking to sponsor for U.S. citizenship. Most recently, the young women had been teaching English as a second language at the University.

Helena was originally from Brazil and was fluent in five languages. She also had a black cocker spaniel named Alex, whom she had with her as a constant companion. She told me he had saved her from depression and suicide at one time by telling her, "You can't leave me behind." She had been in vet school in Brazil, but was too kind-hearted for a livestock-dominated vet program. Her father had been angry over her failure, causing her to move to the U.S. The plan for her citizenship was for the young woman to work for me as an editor for my writing, which she would fund. She also hired an immigration attorney to gain her green card and provided her room and board in an apartment behind my clinic.

Unfortunately, after a couple years with us both trying to help her, she moved in with a boyfriend. From that point, I assume, she became an illegal immigrant. Of course, we were both very disappointed, but the overall experience gave me a lot of insight into the immigration issue. I learned the immigration process done legally is expensive and difficult.

Another area I learned about from this relationship was animal law, animal rights, and animal welfare. For example, animal laws originally come from our Biblical laws, which consider animals as property. Therefore, we've had limited litigation in personal judgements in veterinary medicine since it is defined only by the value of the animal.

Most recently, there has been a strong effort to broaden this definition to include emotional value. This is the result of increased emphasis on the human-animal bond and the higher cost of medical care. Lawyers have seen this as the newest potential market for malpractice judgements. Certainly, in my career, I know my clients do value their pets as family members, but I hope we will never follow in the footsteps of human medicine. Most of my human doctor friends are

unhappy because of their lost freedoms and higher liability insurance costs.

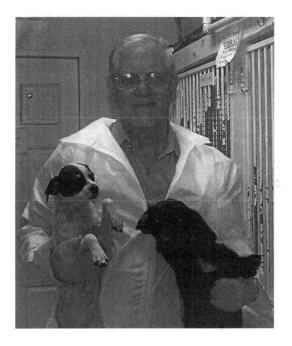

2010 Puerto Rico Humane Society Rescue Operation

Key West Cats

One of my memories goes back to when my wife and I
were flying small airplanes. We had decided to take a
trip to Key West. I was taking no chances since I had
never flown over water. So, I invited a friend who was
a commercial pilot to go with us. One of the traditional
spots to see in Key West is author Earnest Hemmingway's home grounds. He wrote several books while

living in Key West. His home had a beautiful garden with a unique collection of multi-toed cats. Normal cats have five digits, but many of his cat had many more. They are called polydactyl cats. To own a Hemmingway polydactyl cat was highly desired, so they kept a long list of people who wanted to adopt one of their offspring. I decided being a veterinarian, I would take one of the sick ones back with me. However, when I put the cat in the cockpit of the plane, the cat heard the noisy plane engine and went bonkers so I had to take him back.

A Pet Wedding

My final story has pictures to prove the event.

One day, a client brought a small shih tzu named Alex into my clinic for neutering. One of her friends, Barbara, was there at the same time and after finding out about Alex's' surgery appointment. She protested and convinced her friend to cancel the surgery so they could breed him with her shih tzu, Sushi.

Barbara had always been an animal person, often being a surrogate mother to many puppies and kittens over the many years I had known her. She had a menagerie of her own pets and would foster any stray. At her home, she had a flower business which she operated from her garage. Her floral arrangements were the highlight of many of our community's weddings and social events. Later on the day of the spay, when

Barbara got home, the young neighborhood girls that helped her with her animals and her home flower business were told of the plans for breeding the dogs. Apparently, they reminded her that the dogs could not have puppies without being married.

Soon afterwards, Barbara approached me with an unusual request. She asked me if I would officiate in a neighborhood marriage ceremony between Sushi and Alex. The original plan was to have the wedding on a Saturday, but it rained that day. Sunday turned out to be a perfect, sun-drenched Florida afternoon. In attendance for the ceremony were all of the neighborhood parents and grandparents of the bridesmaids, along with the parents of the bride and groom. The scene was in Barbara's beautiful rose garden overlooking a backyard lake. Barbara's husband, a retired judge, constructed a floral archway supported by his fishing rods. Alex, the groom, was handsomely dressed wearing a boutonniere. The bride, Sushi, wore a lace veil and a lovely dress. In the processional, there were nine beautiful 8-10 year-old bridesmaids dressed in their Sunday best. The event was only marred by the groom lifting his leg several times on the way to the alter.

I am a sub-deacon and lay minister in my church, but I was not sure that qualified me for this official duty. However, I gladly accepted. My experience in religion was that different church leaders have different opinions as to an animal's place in God's plan. But as for me, and my theology, my homily went something like this. In the beginning of the Bible creation story, God created the animals first as man's companions and asked him to name them. I have always thought Adam gave the name to dogs, which is God spelled backwards, because they express unconditional love. Later, in the Biblical story of Noah, God recreated the earth by protecting Noah's family and two of all the animals from a great flood.

That day, I told the young girls that just like they witnessed in the union of the two dogs, Alex and Sushi, I hoped each of them would someday find a husband that would give them unconditional love like dogs exhibit. I also told them if it was God's will for them, that they could have babies of their own. I pointed out how much family love was represented that day through our group of neighbors, parents, and grandparents. In that hopeful spirit, I blessed the union of Alex and Sushi, which was followed by a photo shoot and a luncheon for the adults. The young ladies had a tea party where they practiced their social graces. The story had a happy ending because Sushi had four cute, little puppies shortly thereafter. One was even named Bruce. I tried not to show him partiality.

My Faith in Practice as a Veterinarian

ONE OF THE HARDEST parts of being a veterinarian has been in my responsibility to euthanize animals. Before vet school, I never gave much thought to this practice. However, this is the biggest difference in my profession and that of human medicine.

I remember when I started my first job in Miami and the racing greyhound trainers would bring six or more healthy dogs in for euthanasia. Only one or two were kept as blood donors, while the rest were euthanized. A local newspaper wrote an article called, *Run for Your Life*, which told of this tragedy. Thousands of dogs were euthanized just because they were not fast enough. As mentioned in this book, the average greyhound is bred and trained to start racing at about two years of age. As veterinarians, we only treated the best A and B grade dogs, meaning if they did not win or place in their first six races, they were euthanized. I remember asking Dr. Yarborough, my boss at the time, if we could spare some and find them homes. He replied emphatically, "If they tell you to put them to sleep, do it!" That was the price we paid to take care of the faster, more valuable kennel dogs.

From my early farm experiences, humane treatment of animals was another learning experience for me when transitioning to a small animal practice. Now, the love of animals seems to be the motivation for students to attend veterinary school.

I remember in veterinary school that I had a job in a biology lab where stray cats were collected as teaching specimens for an anatomy class. They were inhumanely euthanized by putting a mask over their heads and using asphyxiation with natural gas to euthanize them. I quit that job right away.

Later in my career, I served on the IACUC research hospital committee, where we reviewed protocol for animal research. My responsibility was to check on the humane treatment of animals like ferrets and pigs being used for student education. Surprisingly, I noted occasions where pain control and lack of humane practices while using these animals occurred.

However, when I went to vet school, farm animals were operated on routinely without anesthesia or pain control. Only in recent years has pain management been considered routine in the small animal field.

You might recall my story of attorney and animal activist, Dr. Florence Dunbar, who taught me a lot on the subject of animal rights. All law is based on Biblical law of humane compassionate care of animals.

At another point in my career, I decided to study how I could share my Christian faith in support of my clients before and after the euthanasia of their family pet. After the tragic practice breakup at Howell Branch Animal Hospital, my church community was the first to support me in my rebuilding my new practice. Our church had a program called "Walking the Mourners Path," which I wanted for my pet clients, too. I took a training which taught me pastoral care and grief counseling – neither of which I had been given in vet school. I also started a "Pet Ministry Group," that provided grief support for animal lovers.

In my practice, I would offer a prayer following euthanasia, if appropriate. I would usually include a thanksgiving for the pet's life and memories and ask forgiveness for our taking of life. I offered the client assurance that euthanasia is a final act of love and would encourage them in knowing that it is our Biblical responsibility to prevent suffering in God's creatures.

As I continued to explore my faith in animal practice, I started reading how other religions of the world look at animals, the afterlife, and spirituality. I found that most believed in a god and in their responsibility for the kind and compassionate care of animals. Some believed in an afterlife, like Egyptians and Hindus. As for Christians, I found that in the Eastern Catholic tradition, especially St. Francis of Assisi and the Celtic tradition, they believed that God could be found throughout creation, both in nature and the animal kingdom.

Since I was interested in spirituality, one of my Jewish clients suggested I take a course on the Kabbalah, which explains their belief in souls. They believe there are three types of souls. The angel soul cannot elevate or diminish its position in their relationship to God. They are servants and messengers in God's kingdom. The second type of souls are the animal souls who are like the angels in their relationship. They are sometimes referred to as earthly angels. The third type is man's soul, which can elevate or lower in God's relationship by our actions on earth.

Soul is made up of a combination of our intellect, our emotions, and our will. A good metaphor for soul is light. It never changes, cannot be denied, cannot be felt, spreads instantly, and is essential to life. A candle is light for one's soul when they die. The body being the candle and the flame, the spirit. The spirit controls the soul. The soul controls come from thinking, which controls our brain, including both our consciousness and non-consciousness. Our free will influences our brain and our brains are wired for love. The body, then, carries out the will of the spirit and the soul.

The spirit gives humans a consciousness for God. It alerts us to our need for God, reconciliation, and redemption. This sets us apart from animals who do not need those things and are innocent creatures. We sense our need for God, and he loves us. Thus, I believe animals will be in heaven.

I have read that most people believe they are spiritual, which means something different to each of us. For me, the Holy Spirit gives me a consciousness for God. It alerts me to the need for God, reconciliation, and redemption. This sets us apart from animals who do not need these things and are innocent creatures. We sense our need for God, and he loves us.

I have concluded that children and animals are kindred spirits in that they both share innocence, trust, and unconditional love as common virtues. In the Bible, we are told to be child-like. I think animals can also teach us that God is love and He loves us. The happiness we enjoy with our pets is what God want for us. As it states in Isaiah's Biblical prophecy, animals will be a part of God's peaceful Kingdom to come.

As a child, I never knew about the animal-human bond. One of the first time I witnessed this human animal bond was with a female client I had who would chew food for her beloved chihuahua since the dog had no teeth. The AVMA defines this bond as a beneficial and dynamic relationship between people and their animals. It is influenced by behaviors that are essential to the health and well-being of humans and animals. This bond is important for the emotional, psychological, and physical interactions of people with other animals and their environment. It is relationship like the human-to-human relational connection of love and intimacy.

I personally believe the human-animal bond at its best is characterized by unconditional love. It is a spiritual relationship. I have read that spirit is of tremendous importance to both man and animal. Spirit is Latin for breath and Greek for soul. Spirituality can include a sense of interconnectedness with all living creatures and an awareness of the purpose and meaning of life, including hope, inner peace, and the development of personal absolute values. Acts of compassion and selflessness are characteristics of a spiritual person. Contributions to good spirituality are faith, forgiveness, love, social support, and prayer. Spirit is a critical element in the well-being of a person.

Considering the subject of animal spirituality, I am inclined to reference the "Best Friends Animal Sanctuary" in Utah, which is animal lover's paradise. About 1600 animals call this Sanctuary home. It houses dogs, cats, bunnies, birds, horses, pigs, and other barnyard animals. In this Utah sanctuary, they celebrate the spirituality of our relationship with animals. At a place called Angel Rest, which was once an old American Indian burial ground, they have an animal burial ground.

Biophilia ("friend of life"), developed by biologist E. O. Wilson, ascertains that, *"Humans have a long held psychological need for a relationship with different aspects of the natural world: animal, plants, landscape and wilderness."* For instance, more people go to zoos in our country than all other spectator sports events combined.

From my experience in Miami, I learned that the goals I had to pursue a high level of professional standards by being an AAHA member required annual inspection of my practices above state requirements. Also, Yarborough's example of community activity in Kiwanis Club led me to pursue 20 years of membership in Rotary Club and volunteering in schools for pre-vet education and greyhound rescue program.

Another community organization I have been involved in since boyhood is the YMCA. Starting as a camp counselor to now serving as a board member, I have been involved in the Christian Awareness committee now called the Mission committee. This represents what I believe about faith in Christ, regular exercise, youth and adult sports activities, scholarships, and the character building of youth in Christian values.

One of my proudest accomplishments in my professional career was organizing the original group of vets and securing the property for the first Vet Emergency Clinic in Central Florida. This is now a co-op that now has over a hundred clinics in four locations.

Lastly, as I reflect on the course of my career, I have a lot of people to thank. First, my wife, Barbara, for her constant support and love. Also, her mother, Machen, and Uncle Roy who loved me and supported me in the early days in Crossett. My spiritual father and brother, Frank Temple, who mentored me through my early Christian years and encouraged my use of the Bible, and Oswald Chambers, for being a spiritual guide for so many years. My children, Bryce and Lisa, who have been a blessing to me along with their children. My siblings Bob, Don, Diane who have always supported me also with their love. Our best friends in Nebraska, Randy and Nancy, who have shared so many fond trips and are just like family to us. I have been blessed with other fellow brothers and sisters over the years. There are too many to mention. I only hope to finish my faith journey well, and I thank the Lord for that answered prayer to become a veterinarian so many years ago.